Homemade Body Butters

Look Younger, Healthier and Naturally More Beautiful with these Natural Concoctions

Contents

Introduction

What you slather on your skin matters. The truth is, with the commercially available body butter you are using now, you cannot always be sure whether you are protecting your skin, or causing more harm. The question is this: would you risk using commercial skin products laden with synthetic chemicals or would you rather use home-made body butter made from natural ingredients that would not harm your skin?

This book aims to help you find better, safer and more natural ways to moisturize, rejuvenate and protect your skin so you can look younger and radiant.

The body butter recipes in this book will address some of the most common skin problems that women face today. Here's a quick overview of what awaits you.

Does your skin feel rough and dry? We have 5 of the most nourishing homemade body butter recipes that will surely make your skin feel softer and sexier!

Are you stressed out? Do you feel like you are all worn out? There are body butter recipes that are meant to calm your mind and spirit as well as heal your skin so you feel rejuvenated.

Does the sun bother you a lot? If you are a woman whose lifestyle or job requires going outdoors all the time, you will need body butter with sun-protection properties. Fear the sun no more and show off your amazing skin!

Do you feel like your skin could use a little life? Reveal younger looking skin with our anti-aging body butter concoctions!

Look and feel at your best with the top 25 Homemade Body Butter Recipes in this book.

Chapter 1 – The 5 Most Nourishing Body Butter Recipes

Put an end to dry, rough skin with these moisturizing body butter recipes with ingredients that are easily absorbed by the skin to keep it young and healthy-looking.

Chamomile Body Butter

The scent of chamomile is not only soothing and invigorating; it also has a calming effect. When partnered with nourishing oils, what you get is a moisturizing remedy that can definitely put you in a good mood. This body butter recipe can soften and rejuvenate tired, dry skin.

Ingredients:

- 15 drops of Wild Chamomile essential oil

- Half a teaspoon of vitamin E

- 5 grams of glycerine

- 11 grams of beeswax

- 20 grams of Aloe Vera gel

- 40 grams rosewater

- 60 grams of herb infused oil

Combine the glycerine, aloe vera and rosewater in a small glass cup. In the meantime, place the beeswax in a double boiler to melt. Pour in the infused oil to the mixture. Heat the mixture until the ingredients have melted. Set it aside to cool down to 100 degrees Fahrenheit.

Next, heat the glycerine, aloe vera and rosewater to 100 degrees Fahrenheit then mix with the melted wax using a low speed hand mixer. Pour the melted beeswax and infused oil little by little as you continue to blend the mixture.

Continue blending for 5 more minutes or until the mixture has become creamy and firm like a thick pudding. Transfer into a sterile container and place in the freezer for a couple of hours for the body butter to set.

Hemp and Shea Body Butter

A simple and easy recipe, this body butter features moisturizing ingredients that are easily absorbed by the skin. It will leave your skin feeling soft, silky and absolutely sexy. This body butter can be used for the body, hands and even the face.

Ingredients:

- 15 drops of Frankincense CO2 or Essential Oil

- Two tablespoons of Shea butter

- Two tablespoons of mango butter

- One tablespoon of Hemp seed oil

- One tablespoon of meadowfoam seed oil

- One teaspoon of vitamin E oil

Directions:

In a small mixing bowl, combine the mango and shea butter. Pour in the hemp seed, meadowfoam seed and vitamin E oil. Using a hand-held mixer, blend all the ingredients. Set the mixer on medium high speed and keep mixing for 5 minutes.

Then, add the Frankincense CO2 or Essential oil. Mix again for at least 5 more minutes or until the mixture is thick and creamy. Finally, transfer the mixture in a sanitized container. Store the body butter at room temperature; it will last for four months.

Lavender Body Butter Concoction

This recipe is a perfect solution for a stressed mind and dry skin. The combination of kukui nut oil and shea butter isn't only soothing, but the high penetrability of these ingredients makes it rich in nourishing properties. The added lavender essential oil makes this concoction great for the skin, body and mind as it offers relaxing effects.

Ingredients:

- 50 drops of Lavender Essential oil
- 2 ml of Vitamin E oil
- 7 grams of Stearic Acid
- 10 grams of Beeswax
- 26 grams of Vegetable Glycerine
- 42 grams of Shea Butter
- 56 grams of Aloe Vera Gel
- 72 grams of Kukui Nut Oil

Directions:

Combine the aloe vera gel with the glycerine in a small glass cup. On a separate larger glass cup, mix the kukui nut oil, Shea butter, beeswax and stearic acid together. Heat the larger glass cup until the mixture is fully melted. Set it aside to warm up to at least 120 degrees Fahrenheit. Heat the small glass cup to reach the same temperature.

With both mixtures at 120 degrees Fahrenheit, slowly add the glycerine and aloe vera mixture to the larger glass cup. Mix the contents using a hand held mixer. Turn the mixer up to medium high speed and whisk for about 15 minutes.

Add the vitamin E and essential oil in the mixture. Blend them for a few more minutes. At this point, the texture is thick but is still pourable. To complete the process, transfer the mixture in a sterilized container and refrigerate for a couple of hours to achieve the desired consistency.

Minty Shea Body Butter

This is a luxurious body butter recipe. It moisturizes the skin well and the ingredients penetrate the skin easily too for a long lasting effect. The Kukui nut oil ingredient of this homemade body butter recipe is rich in essential fatty acids, alpha-linolenic and linoleic acid. These fatty acids help maintain a healthy complexion to improve skin texture and make it feel softer.

It is soothing for chapped and dry skin. It is also great for sensitive skin and can even serve as a remedy for psoriasis and eczema. The addition of rosemary and spearmint essential oils provide this Shea body butter a fragrant and minty aroma, which can make you feel refreshed and revitalized.

Ingredients:

90 grams of Shea butter

45 grams of Cocoa butter

45 grams of Kukui nut oil

10 drops of Rosemary oil

20 drops of Spearmint oil

Directions:

Mix the cocoa butter with the Shea butter in a medium metal bowl or glass bowl. Pour in the Kukui nut oil. Put the bowl over a small pan containing simmering water on low heat. This should make the butters and oil melt. This may take around 5 minutes.

Once the butter and oil have melted, set the mixture aside to cool. After 10 minutes, place the bowl with the melted ingredients in the fridge. Let it stay inside for about 20 minutes.

After 20 minutes, take the bowl out. Using a whisk attachment, blend the mixture for 5 minutes. Then, put it back in the fridge and let it stay there for 15 minutes or more. Take it out of the fridge and whisk again until the mixture turns into a creamy color. Place it back in the fridge.

When the mixture becomes super cold, take it out again and whisk. Scoop the sides of the bowl and pour the essential oils. Blend again and transfer in a container. This body butter recipe can last up to 60 days as long as you keep it cool. Make sure you also store it in a cool, dark place.

Rosy Coconut Body Butter

Coconut oil has so many uses in itself. However, this body butter recipe will turn your dry skin all the way around to healthy, nourished skin. With coconut oil as the main moisturizing agent, adding a bit of corn-starch to it will leave your skin without an oily feel. Since this recipe is loaded with rose essential oil and jojoba oil, you can be sure it will make your skin smelling fresh while leaving it hydrated.

Ingredients:

- 10 drops of Rose essential oil

- 3 grams of cornstarch

- 10 grams of Jojoba oil

- 60 grams of refined coconut oil

Directions:

Mix the jojoba oil, coconut oil and cornstarch together in a glass bowl. Place the bowl in a pan with simmering water to melt the coconut oil. Whisk the ingredients well and set aside to cool.

When cooled, pour the rose essential oil into the mixture. Whisk again until it becomes fluffy like a frosting. Transfer in a small jar and keep refrigerated. This lasts up to 3 months.

Chapter 2 – Top 5 Soothing Body Butter Recipes

If you are feeling stressed, it will show. Body butter can also be used to soothe tired and worn out skin. The following homemade recipes can help refresh and heal sore skin.

Aloe Body Butter

Aloe Vera has been used for numerous things by itself, and if you start making your own body butter recipe with it as the main ingredient, you will regret ever using commercially produced body butter. This next recipe isn't only used to soothe and nourish your skin, but it can also be used to treat sun burns, scars, acne and more. What more can you ask for?

Ingredients:

- Three tablespoons of Aloe Vera
- Three tablespoons of Shea Butter
- Two tablespoons of Coconut oil
- One tablespoon of Avocado Oil
- One tablespoon of Vitamin E oil
- 10 to 15 drops of your preferred essential oil

Directions:

First, melt the Shea butter and coconut oil in a double boiler. Once fully melted, remove the mixture from the heat and set aside to cool until it appears opaque.

Next, pour in the rest of the ingredients and mix using a hand mixer for 5 to 10 minutes. You know the body butter is ready when it has become light, fluffy and thick enough to stick to a spoon that is held upside down.

Transfer the mixture into a sterilized small container and place in the refrigerator.

Blossoming Body Butter

The cocoa, Shea butter and coconut oil in this body recipe provide a hydrating effect while the essential oils help regenerate and rejuvenate your skin while calming your mind.

Ingredients:

- 6 drops of Frankincense essential oil
- 6 drops of Neroli essential oil
- 8 drops of Lavender essential oil
- 5 grams of Evening Primrose oil
- 5 grams of Peach kernel oil
- 10 grams of unrefined coconut oil
- 10 grams of Cocoa butter
- 20 grams of Jojoba oil
- 50 grams of Shea butter

Directions:

First, melt the Shea butter and cocoa butter in a double boiler. Once melted, set it aside to cool.

As the butter mixture cools, add the essential oils. Mix thoroughly using a low speed hand mixer until light and fluffy.

When the mixture starts to solidify, transfer into a small sterilized container and store in the refrigerator.

Calming Lavender Body Butter

This body butter recipe combines the moisturizing Shea butter and coconut oil with the soothing marshmallow root and calendula.

Ingredients:

- Three fourth cup of unrefined Shea butter

- Quarter cup of extra virgin coconut oil

- Two tablespoons of dried marshmallow root

- Two tablespoons of calendula petals

- Eight drops of peppermint essential oil

- Eight drops of lavender essential oil

Directions:

First, preheat the oven to 200 degrees. Then, turn it off after 5 minutes. In a small pan, melt the shea butter and coconut oil. Once melted, add the herbs into the mix. Stir and put the pan inside the oven.

Leave it inside for 4 hours or more to allow the herbs to steep. Next, separate the oil from the herbs using a fine strainer.

Add the infused oil, and then put it inside the fridge to cool. Before the mixture solidifies, take it out and whip using a hand held mixer for 30 seconds or more. Pour in the essential oils and mix again for about a minute or so.

Transfer in a small glass container and store in the refrigerator.

This body butter is best used at night. Apply it at least half an hour before you go to bed.

Simply Soothing Whipped Body Butter

Tamanu oil has antioxidant, antibacterial and anti-inflammatory properties. This is a tropical oil that will help repair damaged skin. The coconut and Frankincense oils further enhance the relief felt from exhaustion, stress and tension in your body. This recipe will make you feel rested and relaxed that you would want to use this every time you may be stressed out.

Ingredients:

- One cup of coconut oil

- One and a half teaspoon of tamanu oil

- A couple drops of Frankincense oil

Directions:

Using a mixer, blend all the ingredients together for about 5 minutes or until it has become light and fluffy. Transfer into a glass container and store in the refrigerator. This simple body butter is ready for use anytime, anywhere.

Soothing Coffee Body Butter

Do you stand all day that your feet start to ache, but you don't know what to do? Well, this is it. This recipe is a great remedy for tired feet. The delicious aroma of the coffee butter along with peppermint and chocolate fragrances will make this recipe an indulgent treat. It is best used before going to bed. For best results, cover your feet with socks after application.

Ingredients:

- 0.7 ounce of White Beeswax

- 1 ounce of Emulsifying Wax

- 1.2 ounces of Stearic Acid

- 2.4 ounces of Sunflower Oil

- 3.1 ounces of Coffee Butter

- 15.6 ounces of Distilled Water

- 5 ml of Peppermint 2nd Distillation Essential Oil

- 5 ml of Dark Rich Chocolate Fragrance Oil

Directions:

Melt the coffee butter, emulsifying wax, beeswax, stearic acid and sunflower oil in a glass jar. You can place it in a small pan with simmering water or melt in the microwave.

Then, heat the distilled water in a separate container up to 150 to 155 degrees Fahrenheit. The oil mixture and the water must be in the same temperature.

Blend them together continuously for at least 2 or 3 minutes. Set the mixture aside to cool down. When it has cooled, add in the essential and fragrance oil. Continue blending for about a minute or two.

Transfer in a sterilized container. Let it cool then put on the lid and store in the refrigerator.

Chapter 3 – 5 Body Butter Blends For Sun Protection

What do you use to keep your face and skin protected from UV rays? Sun protection is important for everyone. To keep your skin looking fresh, feeling soft and healthy, adequate sun protection is needed. Making one or all of the recipes below will provide you with a natural, sun-protecting concoction while keeping your skin moisturized.

Bee Sun Protected

With only four ingredients, this incredible recipe provides natural protection against sun damage. Not only does it protect from UV rays, but it also moisturizes your skin to maintain a healthier glow.

Ingredients:

- Half an ounce of beeswax

- Quarter cup of coconut oil

- Quarter cup of Shea butter

- Two tablespoons of zinc oxide powder

Directions:

Combine the coconut oil with the beeswax and the Shea butter. Melt them and set aside. When the mixture has cooled a bit, drizzle in the zinc oxide powder. Then, take a handheld mixer. Whisk the mixture until there are no more clumps from the zinc oxide powder. Now transfer the mixture into a glass mason jar. Let it cool to room temperature before storing in the fridge.

Sun Blocking Body Butter

Did you know that SPF (sun protection factor) is referred to as the ability of a sunblock or sunscreen to block UVB rays? If you didn't, now you do! This recipe has SPF 40 that blocks UVB rays and protects your skin from sun damage and sunburn.

Ingredients:

- Two tablespoons of coconut oil

- One tablespoon of avocado oil

- One tablespoon of Shea butter

- Half a teaspoon of aloe Vera gel

- Half a teaspoon of sesame oil

- Thirty drops of carrot seed oil

Directions:

Start by melting the Shea butter and coconut oil using a double boiler. Once melted, let it cool down to room temperature for a couple of minutes.

Stir in the rest of the ingredients. Whisk gently.

Before the mixture solidifies, transfer in a glass jar. Store it in a cool and dry place. Use as necessary.

Sunscreen Shea Body Butter

Shea butter is known for its moisturizing effect, but it also has natural sun protection properties, providing SPF 4 to 5 from its Vitamins E and F content. With the addition of Zinc Oxide, this body butter recipe is great for protecting your skin against sun damage. Overall, this body butter provides SPF 30.

Ingredients:

- One cup of Shea butter

- Half a cup of Olive oil

- Half a cup of Coconut oil

- Three tablespoons of Zinc Oxide powder

- Two tablespoons of liquid Vitamin E

- Four ounces of beeswax

Directions:

Mix all the ingredients in a crock pot, but leave the Zinc Oxide powder out. Heat until everything in the pot has fully melted. Slowly stir in the Zinc Oxide powder. Whisk gently. While the mixture is still liquid, transfer in a glass container. Set it aside to cool. Once it is cool enough, put inside the fridge.

Sunscreen Body Cream

This body cream contains titanium dioxide that completely blocks UVA and UVB short rays from the sun. The beeswax, on the other hand, helps prolong the sun protecting ability of this body butter while the eucalyptus oil further enhances the effects of the other ingredients.

Ingredients:

- 200 ml of coconut oil
- 120 ml of cocoa butter
- 120 ml of Shea butter
- 60 ml of beeswax
- Six tablespoons of titanium dioxide
- Fifteen drops of eucalyptus oil

Directions:

Combine the cocoa butter and beeswax in a double boiler to melt. Mix in the coconut oil and Shea butter. Once melted and mixed, remove the mixture from heat and let it cool to body temperature.

Once cooled, stir in the eucalyptus oil. Mix well. Gradually add the titanium dioxide. Stir the mixture using a handheld mixer at low speed until it becomes light and fluffy.

Set aside for a couple of hours and you will get a heavier and harder cream you can use before heading to the beach.

Sun Protecting Butter

You should already know by now that body butter helps rejuvenate your skin. However, this recipe protects you and your skin from the sun. Beyond that, it also helps you smell sweet and fresh with the essential oils used. Moreover, all the ingredients combined boost the sunscreen effect.

Ingredients:

- 90 ml of unrefined vegetable oil or a combination of avocado, flaxseed, palm, coconut, canola, sunflower and olive oil

- 90 ml of distilled water

- 60 ml of Shea butter

- 30 ml of cocoa butter

- Two tablespoons of walnut oil

- Two tablespoons of titanium dioxide powder

- Two tablespoons of calendula oil

- Ten drops of lavender oil

- Three drops of vanilla oil

- Three drops of mint oil

Directions:

Start by melting the cocoa and Shea butter in a double boiler. Once melted, set it aside to cool.

In the meantime, mix the vegetable oil with the walnut and calendula oil. Combine it with the melted mixture. When the mixture has cooled down, stir in the lavender essential oil along with the mint and vanilla essential oils.

Take a dark glass container and pour in the zinc oxide and titanium dioxide. Next, add the distilled water and pour in the oil mixture. Make sure that all the ingredients are of the same temperature as you mix them. Store in the fridge and shake well before each use.

Chapter 4 – Top 5 Anti-Aging Body Butter Recipes

Are you worried about looking older? Try out these body butter recipes that may help you beat the hands of time!

Cellulite Busting Cinnamon Butter

The star of this body butter recipe is the skin firming cinnamon. Rich in calcium, iron and magnesium, cinnamon improves blood circulation and rids off cellulite.

Ingredients:

Cinnamon stick

Thirty drops of cinnamon oil

Fifty grams of Shea butter

Fifty grams of cocoa butter

A Hundred grams of coconut oil

Directions:

Melt the Shea and coconut butter in a small pan over low heat. Stir in the coconut oil gradually. Stir for a minute and remove the pan from the heat. Set aside to cool for 10 to 20 minutes.

As the mixture cools, pour in the cinnamon oil. Whisk the mixture with a hand held mixer until it is light and fluffy. Break the cinnamon sticks into small pieces and add to the mixture.

Transfer in a glass container and store in a cool and dry place.

Honey Citrus Butter

Honey and lemon are used so many things, so why not use it for your skin? This recipe utilizes these two versatile ingredients to help increase the skin's elasticity and treat unwanted wrinkles naturally.

Ingredients:

- Half a cup of Grapeseed oil

- Two tablespoons of beeswax

- Two tablespoons of distilled water

- One capsule of vitamin E oil

- Ten drops of lemon essential oil

Directions:

Mix the beeswax with the vitamin E oil and Grapeseed oil in a Pyrex container. Heat the ingredients in the microwave until fully melted and mixed.

Use a hand mixer to whip the oils then add distilled water gradually. Keep whipping until the mixture is milky. Next, stir in the essential oil and whip a little more. Set it aside to settle.

Once the mixture has set, transfer into a glass mason jar. Refrigerate and it is ready for use.

Skin Firming Body Butter

This body butter's waxy texture waterproofs and lubricates the skin to make it soft, supple and younger looking.

Ingredients:

- One cup of Shea butter

- Half a cup of jojoba oil

- Half a cup of tallow

- Two teaspoons of vitamin E oil

- One teaspoon of peppermint essential oil

Directions:

Gently heat the tallow and Shea butter in a double boiler. Once melted, remove the mixture from the heat and add the jojoba oil. Set aside to cool.

Once the mixture has cooled down, pour the vitamin E oil along with the essential oil. Stir well. Then, continue to chill the mixture in the fridge.

Take it out after 5 to 10 minutes and whip using a hand mixer until light and fluffy. Transfer in a mason jar and refrigerate.

Regenerating Shea Butter

Are you stressed from work? Or do you stay up all night? This recipe fights and eliminates fine lines and wrinkles that add years to your skin. But why stop there when this recipe also helps eliminate unwanted scars while leaving your skin rejuvenated and smell amazing?

Ingredients:

- One cup of raw Shea butter

- Half a cup of coconut oil

- Quarter a cup of almond oil

- Half a teaspoon of vitamin E oil

Directions:

Heat the coconut oil and Shea butter to melt using a double boiler. Set aside to cool down to room temperature.

Next, stir in the vitamin E and almond oil. Place the mixture in the fridge for about half to one hour.

Mix using a handheld mixer until thick and fluffy. Transfer in a mason jar and refrigerate.

Rejuvenating Body Butter

The combination of the ingredients in this body butter makes a perfect healing agent for stretch marks, scar tissue and dermatitis.

Ingredients:

- Half a cup of Shea butter

- Half a cup of cocoa butter

- Ten ml of Rosehip oil

- Five ml of Argan oil

- Twenty drops of vanilla extract

- Ten drops of Frankincense

Directions:

Melt the Shea and cacao butter in a double boiler. Once melted, remove from heat and stir in the oils and vanilla extract. Use a handheld mixer for blending the ingredients.

Transfer the mixture in a glass container. Store it in the fridge to fully set.

This body butter is best used after a shower.

Chapter 5 – 5 All-Around Body Butter

If you want a little more from your homemade body butter than to merely moisturize, simply soothe or just protect you from the sun, then you've got to try these body butter recipes to get two or more benefits in one cream.

Aloe Butter

Are pimples and acne bothering you? Enriched with aloe Vera, lanolin, beeswax and other natural ingredients, this body butter can also help enhance blood circulation as well as condition and tone the skin.

Ingredients:

- One vitamin E capsule

- Four tablespoons of coconut oil

- Three tablespoons of aloe Vera gel

- Two tablespoons of beeswax

- One and a half tablespoons of olive oil

- Two teaspoons of lanolin

- One teaspoon of honey

- Ten drops of lavender essential oil

Directions:

Heat the beeswax along with the honey, coconut and olive oils in a double boiler over medium heat to melt. Once the ingredients are fully melted, remove from heat and set aside.

Heat the aloe Vera on a separate boiler. Then, add in the beeswax mixture. Stir in the lanolin. Mix well. And reduce the heat to low.

Next, add the contents of the vitamin E capsule along with the lavender essential oil. Mix until you reach a smooth texture.

Remove from heat and transfer in a small glass container. Let it cool to room temperature before sealing and storing in the fridge. When the mixture has fully settled, this body butter is ready for use.

Chocolate Body Butter

Aside from being edible, this recipe also serves as food for your skin. The cocoa butter and coconut oil provide a detoxifying and nourishing effect while the essential oils can make you feel more relaxed. But what makes this body butter special is its sensual effect. It contains cistanche and maca which are known to promote sexual prowess.

Ingredients:

- Three fourth cup of melted coconut oil

- One third cup of clear agave nectar

- Quarter cup of cacao powder

- Half a tablespoon of vanilla powder

- One teaspoon of maca powder

- Half a teaspoon cistanche

- Half a teaspoon of powdered lavender flowers

- Two drops of rose essential oil

Directions:

Blend all the ingredients in a food processor. Process until well blended. Transfer in a small jar and seal. Store it in the fridge for the mixture to fully set. Save this body butter for special occasions.

Magnesium Butter

This body butter homemade recipe does not only make your skin look and feel healthy. It can also provide you adequate sun and UV protection. Magnesium oil makes the skin soft and silky while the Shea butter and coconut oil provide natural SPF for protection.

It also provides a soothing power to relieve sore muscles. Aside from nourishing and protecting your skin, magnesium body butter can enhance your sleep. It also helps when you need that extra boost of magnesium in your body.

Ingredients:

- Half a cup of Magnesium Flakes

- Three tablespoons of boiling water

- Quarter cup of unrefined coconut oil

- Three tablespoons of Shea Butter

- Two tablespoons of Beeswax Pastilles

Directions:

Combine the magnesium flakes with the three tablespoons of boiling water in a small container. Stir the mixture until the magnesium flakes are well dissolved. This will produce a thick consistency. Leave it aside and let the mixture cool.

Now, take a mason jar about a quart size, pour in the beeswax, coconut oil and Shea butter. Place the mason jar inside a small pan that has about an inch of water. Put it over medium heat to let the ingredients melt. As soon as the ingredients melt, take the mason jar out of the pan. Put it aside and let it cool.

When the beeswax, coconut oil and Shea butter mixture cools, pour it into a blender. Process it on medium speed until the oil mixture is well blended.

Take the magnesium mixture and pour it one drop at a time into the oil mixture. Once it is well mixed, put the blended mixture in the fridge and let it stay there for at least 15 minutes.

After 15 minutes, take the mixture out of the fridge and blend again until you achieve a body butter consistency. To maintain this consistency, store the magnesium butter in the fridge or at room temperature. This body butter lasts up to two months.

Mango Coconut Body Butter

Besides its antioxidant properties, this body butter is great for the face too! It can help clearing out clogged pores, blackheads, acne and dark spots. In addition to this, it provides deep nourishment and helps to cool the body down.

Ingredients:

- Thirty drops of mango essential oil
- Thirty grams of mango butter
- Thirty grams of coconut oil
- Twenty grams of Shea butter

Directions:

Combine the Shea butter with the coconut oil in a pan over medium heat. Mix the ingredients until fully melted. Gradually add the mango butter and keep stirring for a minute. Remove the pan from the heat and set aside to cool for about 10 to 20 minutes.

As the mixture cools down, stir in the mango essential oil. Using a handheld mixer, whip the mixture until it appears light and fluffy.

Transfer in an air tight glass container. Store it in a cool and dry place.

Vanilla Body Butter

This body butter can deeply moisturize your skin with its skin enhancing ingredients coconut oil and cocoa butter. Fresh vanilla gives it a sensual fragrance that provides a pleasing and relaxing effect on your mind, body and spirit. Use it before going to bed to get a good night's sleep.

Ingredients:

- One Vanilla bean, ground

- One cup of raw cocoa butter

- Half a cup of coconut oil

- Half a cup of sweet almond oil

Directions:

Combine the coconut oil and cocoa butter in a small pan over low heat to melt. Set aside to cool. After 30 minutes, add the vanilla bits and stir in the sweet almond oil into the melted mixture. Blend well and put in the freezer for 20 minutes.

Take the mixture out for some whipping using an electric mixer. Keep whipping until you reach the desired consistency. Transfer in a glass jar and keep refrigerated.

Conclusion

Thank you again for downloading this book!

I hope you enjoyed reading about my book on the 25 best homemade and all natural body butter recipes. The next step is to start trying them out and feel the nourishing, soothing, sun-protecting and anti-aging effects on your skin.

If you enjoyed this book, please take the time to share your thoughts and **post a professional review on Amazon**. It'd be greatly appreciated!

Thank you!

www.ingramcontent.com/pod-product-compliance
Lightning Source LLC
Chambersburg PA
CBHW081808280526
45789CB00008B/3056